DRUGS and ATHLETES

by Dr. Gloria M. Bertacchi, Pharm. D.

NATIONAL MEDICAL SEMINARS, INC.
Roseville, California

NATIONAL MEDICAL SEMINARS, INC.
P.O. Box 2699
Roseville, CA 95746
(916) 784-6200

For information on book distributors and other titles by this author, please write to NATIONAL MEDICAL SEMINARS, INC. at the above address.

DRUGS and ATHLETES

Copyright 1988 by Dr. Gloria M. Bertacchi. All rights reserved. Printed in the U.S.A. No part of this book may be reproduced by any mechanical, photographic or electronic process, or in the form of a phonographic recording, nor may it be stored in a retrieval system, transmitted or otherwise copied for public or private use without written permission of the publisher.

ISBN 0-945753-03-9

Information has been obtained by NATIONAL MEDICAL SEMINARS, INC. from sources believed to be reliable. However, because of the possibility of human or mechanical error by our sources, NATIONAL MEDICAL SEMINARS, INC. or others, NATIONAL MEDICAL SEMINARS, INC. does not guarantee the accuracy, adequacy, or completeness of any information and is not responsible for any errors or omissions or the results obtained from use of such information.

```
615.704 B536a c. 2

Bertacchi, Gloria M.

Drugs and athletes
```

DRUGS and ATHLETES

TABLE OF CONTENTS

I.	INTRODUCTION.	1
II.	ANABOLIC STEROIDS	1
III.	THE STIMULANTS	5
	A. AMPHETAMINES.	5
	B. STIMULANT SUBSTANCES	8
	C. CAFFEINE	9
	D. NICOTINE	11
	E. COCAINE	13
IV.	CANNABINOIDS.	14
V.	BETA BLOCKERS	16
VI.	THE DEPRESSANTS	18
	A. ALCOHOL	18
	B. SEDATIVE-HYPNOTICS	21
	C. THE BENZODIAZEPINES	22
VII.	SKELETAL MUSCLE RELAXANTS . .	24
VIII.	PAIN MEDICATIONS.	24
IX.	ANTI-INFLAMMATORY AGENTS . . .	26
X.	CORTICOSTEROIDS	26
XI.	DIMETHYL SULFOXIDE (DMSO) . . .	27
XII.	BLOOD DOPING.	27
XIII.	MISCELLANEOUS DRUGS OF ABUSE .	28
XIV.	DRUG CONTROL PROGRAMS OF THE OLYMPIC COMMITTEE	30
XV.	IDENTIFYING THE DRUG ABUSER. .	33
XVI.	CASE STUDIES	34
XVII.	CONCLUSION.	38
BIBLIOGRAPHY		40
GLOSSARY.		41

I. **INTRODUCTION**

Drug abuse in the sports world has been prevalent throughout the past thirty years. In 1983 at the Pan American Games, the first accurate laboratory method of drug identification in urine was revealed. Many athletes refused to be tested, resulting in widespread controversy.

The United States Olympic Committee (USOC) and the International Olympic Committee (IOC) currently have a program to detect drug abuse in athletes. The purpose is to determine drug abuse and to disqualify athletes who use drugs during competition.

The reasons that athletes use drugs are to increase their self-assurance, motivation, endurance, and performance. However, athletes seldom realize the true side effects, toxicity, and adverse effects on performance that many drugs exert. Athletes abuse a variety of drugs and substances ranging from oxygen to steroids.

II. **ANABOLIC STEROIDS**

The most common drugs of abuse in the sports world are called anabolic steroids. Anabolic steroids are derived from testosterone, a male hormone. These steroids will cause masculine effects and tissue building.

Anabolic steroids are used as a treatment for testosterone deficiency, anemia, and swelling. Transsexual females use anabolic steroids to develop masculine characteristics.

DRUGS AND ATHLETES

In the early 1950's the Russians used anabolic steroids to increase athletic prowess. It was believed that Germans used anabolic steroids during the war to improve the soldier's aggressiveness. Primarily used to increase strength and muscle size by weight lifters and body builders, anabolic steroids have been used by an array of athletes including runners, swimmers, wrestlers, and football players.

Anabolic steroids disrupt hormones and their feedback system. The hypothalamus in the brain determines the body's requirements for testosterone. Exercise, for example, will decrease the stores of testosterone. This will stimulate testosterone production. This in turn will cause protein synthesis. The hypothalamus will trigger the pituitary gland to manufacture a hormone stimulant, gonadotropin, which will then stimulate production of testosterone.

Interference in this feedback system will stop the production of testosterone. For this reason, anabolic steroids have been considered as a possible future male birth control agent. The size of the testes may actually decrease from the use of anabolic steroids. Also, abnormal sperm cells may result from their use. Therefore, anabolic steroids have yet to be used as a male birth control agent due to these unwarranted side effects.

Due to shut down of testosterone production, estrogen, a female hormone, will be stimulated in the receptors in the body. Therefore, the use of anabolic steroids may trigger the development of male mammary glands. This will appear as small female breasts in which clear fluid may be secreted. Even when anabolic steroids are discontinued, this breast tissue may not disappear. Some anabolic users will take anti-hormone agents such as tamoxifen (Nolvadex) to reverse these effects. Surgical removal of breast tissue has been recommended for patients with this increased breast tissue.

Anabolic steroids may have an effect on sexual performance. Initially the sex drive may increase. However, after several weeks there may actually be a decrease in sexual drive. It is not until steroids are discontinued and at least two weeks have passed allowing the testes to increase their testosterone levels, that the resumption of the sex drive will occur. Some users have stated that their sex drive was never normal after the use of anabolic steroids.

Some of the other side effects that can occur with the use of steroids include increased acne and loss of hair. Users may become aggressive and irritable. They may become more apt to fight or lash out.

Muscle strength may increase faster than the strength of the tissue and tendons, and thus there may be increased injury to the athlete.

Users of anabolic steroids may have a greater long-term risk of heart disease. High blood pressure and heart attacks may occur in users. Liver tumors, hepatitis (viral inflammation of the liver), and blood cyst disorders can result

DRUGS AND ATHLETES

from the use of anabolic steroids. Liver cancer and kidney tumors from anabolic steroid use have caused deaths in athletes.

Anabolic steroids can cause changes in liver tests. However, this does not necessarily indicate liver damage. Other tests may have to be performed to determine whether liver damage has indeed occurred.

Anabolic steroids can be used by mouth or injected into the veins (intravenous). The abuse of intravenous drugs and the sharing of needles can cause the transmission of hepatitis, heart inflammation and AIDS.

Serious problems are seen in women who use anabolic steroids. These women may develop masculine characteristics including excessive hair growth, lowering of the voice, and increased clitoris size. These effects may not be reversible. Other effects including irregular menstruation, decreased sex drive, acne and aggressiveness which may reverse upon discontinuation of these drugs.

There is still controversy concerning anabolic steroids and their effects on muscle mass and strength. It appears that anabolic steroids do increase muscle size and strength but with resultant serious side effects.

III. THE STIMULANTS

A. AMPHETAMINES

Central nervous system stimulants, amphetamines or "uppers" are strictly controlled drugs which are seldom prescribed due to their serious withdrawal and side effects. Amphetamines have been used to treat obesity, paralysis, mental depression, alcohol withdrawal, premenstrual tension, narcolepsy (an uncontrollable desire to sleep), and an abnormal increase in the body's motor function or activity.

Amphetamines are used in the sports world to enhance a player's athletic ability. However, an athlete may injure himself because he feels mentally capable of activities that he physically is unable to accomplish. The athlete will have an increased alertness while using amphetamines. However, each person will have significant and inconsistent reactions to the amphetamines. Therefore, the effects of amphetamines are dependant on the person's bodily function and the person's health status.

Amphetamines will not stop an athlete from becoming fatigued (tired). Amphetamines will, however, cover up the effects of fatigue and interfere with the body's ability to recognize fatigue. This can lead to serious consequences as the athlete feels capable of athletic performance when he is in reality extremely tired.

Athletes will abuse amphetamines not only to relieve tiredness, but also to elevate their mood and increase alertness. Athletes believe that amphetamines will help psyche them up and

DRUGS AND ATHLETES

increase their energy level prior to a competitive performance. The athlete will feel excited, ready to perform, and increasingly eager to enter competition.

Amphetamines will cause an increase in blood pressure, heart rate and metabolic rate. The smooth muscle will be relaxed. For example, there will be a decrease in intestine movement and an increase in breathing. The pupils will widen and salivation will decrease. There will be an increase in oxygen requirements due to the increased breathing. Rapid eye movement dream sleep (REM) will be decreased which will lead to the user's confusion and sight and sound hallucinations.

The onset of action from an oral dose of the amphetamines is one-half to one hour. The physical effects of the amphetamines last from four to twenty-four hours depending upon the type of amphetamine used.

Amphetamines are central nervous system stimulants and cause a variety of adverse effects. Some adverse effects include an increase in anxiety, confusion, inability to sleep and mental illness. Fever and dry mouth may also result. Due to the stimulation of the heart from the increase in norepinephrine, a hormone secreted from the brain, deaths can result from the use of amphetamines. These deaths are normally due to irregular heart beats, greatly increased body temperature, and bleeding of the brain.

Anxious and irritable, the amphetamine

THE STIMULANTS

abuser will have a continual urge to move about or pace the floor. His moods may change dramatically from depression to excitement. Happy, content, and calm one moment, the user may suddenly become hostile, aggressive, and belligerent. Paranoia develops in the chronic user who may resort to violence to protect himself.

There is a tendency to become addicted to the amphetamines. This is complicated by the user's desire to avoid the withdrawal depression and to prolong the amphetamine high. Withdrawal from long-term use of amphetamines results in confusion, nightmares, lethargy, suicidal depression, and hostile behavior. This withdrawal syndrome is usually very severe, especially if continuous high doses are stopped suddenly.

Symptoms of amphetamine overdose include: high blood pressure, increased heart rate, headache, dizziness, tremors, convulsions, fever, and sight and sound hallucinations.

Other drugs in the amphetamine class include Eskatrol, Benzedrine, Dexedrine known as "dexies", Biphetamine known as "Black Beauties", and Phenmetrazine (Preludin).

Methedrine and Desoxyn known on the street as "crank", "crystal", and "meth" contain methamphetamine. Many underground laboratories currently manufacture this popular drug of abuse.

Methylphenidate (Ritalin) is another central nervous system stimulant chemically similar to the amphetamines. Used primarily in hyperkinetic

DRUGS AND ATHLETES

children, the major effects of Ritalin are mental rather than physical stimulation.

The amphetamines, through their stressful effects, can be hazardous and in some cases fatal to the athlete. However, these adverse effects are inconsistent and unpredictable.

B. STIMULANT SUBSTANCES

Many products have been developed to replace amphetamines. Many athletes will use these stimulant substances when amphetamines are not easily obtained. These prescription drugs include benzphetamine (Didrex), chlorphentermine (Pre-State), diethylpropion (Tenuate, Tepanil), mazindol (Sanorex), phendimetrazine (Plegine, Statobex, etc.) and phentermine (Ionamin, Fastin). Although these drugs cause effects similar to the amphetamines, they have less addiction and abuse potential.

Ephedrine, pseudoephedrine (Sudafed), and phenylpropanolamine (Control, Dietac, Diadax, etc.) are over-the-counter products pharmacologically similar to the amphetamines. They are marketed as nasal decongestants and weight loss products.

Rapid pulse, dizziness, headaches, and irregular heart beats may result from use of these prescription or over-the-counter stimulants. These symptoms may indicate a temporary increase in blood pressure. All of the stimulants are subject to abuse by athletes and may aggravate diabetes, high blood pressure and thyroid disorders.

THE STIMULANTS

C. CAFFEINE

Caffeine is a synthetic product derived from the alkaloids Cola acuminata and Coffee arabica. The average American consumes 16 pounds of caffeine annually. Caffeine is found in many beverages including colas, sodas, cocoa, tea, and coffee. Many over-the-counter (OTC) and prescription products including diet aids (i.e. Dexatrim), and pain medications (i.e. APC, or aspirin/ phenacetin/ caffeine) contain caffeine. Chocolate also has concentrations of caffeine.

Caffeine is a compound similar to the anti-asthmatic drug, theophylline. Used by mouth, it takes effect quickly and peak effects occur within an hour. Caffeine has a half-life of 3.5 hours. Metabolism occurs in the liver and is eliminated through the kidneys. Heart rate, metabolic rate, and blood pressure will be stimulated by the use of caffeine.

Stomach acid is stimulated by caffeine. Therefore, caffeine can trigger stomach problems such as ulcers.

Athletes claim that caffeine will increase their endurance and performance and increase their energy level. This is achieved by stimulation of the central nervous system, increased skeletal muscle contraction and breakdown of fatty tissue.

Caffeine will cause fat breakdown and increased levels of fatty acids. These fatty acids will be used as fuel by the athlete. Thus, the

DRUGS AND ATHLETES

muscle carbohydrate stores will not be used or depleted.

Caffeine can cause many adverse effects including shaking, headaches, irritability, increased urination and irregular heartbeats. These effects of the drug result in a state called caffeinism. The primary symptoms that occur include: 1) anxiety attacks, 2) morbid anxiety about one's own health, 3) headaches (including migraine headaches) 4) inability to sleep, 5) depression, and 6) withdrawal symptoms. Other central nervous system effects include an increase in activity, a dryness in the mouth, ringing of the ears, shooting pains, and restlessness.

Caffeine will have heart effects in the muscular substance of the heart. It will cause an increase in heartbeats, the heart's force of contraction, and the heart rate. Caffeine can trigger an increase in heart rate. Therefore removal of caffeine from the diet may be necessary to prevent this condition.

The withdrawal syndrome that can occur among people who use caffeine on a regular basis and in great quantities may include: depression, inability to function, headache, sleepiness, runny nose and anxiety. This withdrawal syndrome can be treated by gradually decreasing the amount of caffeine used.

Caffeine is primarily abused by athletes to increase endurance. It can increase muscle contraction, utilize fat, and eliminate fatigue. However, the adverse effects from caffeine

THE STIMULANTS

including the heart effects (i.e. an increase in heart rate) and the central nervous system effects (i.e. inability to sleep and irritability) may also occur. Caffeine is not allowed by the United States Olympic Committee (USOC) and is banned in amounts greater than 15 micrograms per milliliter as tested in the bloodstream.

D. NICOTINE

Nicotine has a long history of abuse dating back to the American Indians who smoked lobeline which is similar to nicotine. The original inhabitants of Australia chewed leaves which contained a substance similar to nicotine. Rolling and chewing of tobacco became popular in the United States in the late 18th century.

Currently, there has been an increase in the use of "chew" tobacco. Many football and baseball players are popularly using this smokeless tobacco. Statistics indicate there are over twenty million users of smokeless tobacco.

Nearly three quarters of high school seniors have tried nicotine and 20% use it on a regular basis. There has actually been a decline since 1977 in the use of nicotine and cigarette smoking among high school seniors. There appears to be a trend among all ages in decreasing cigarette smoking and nicotine use. However, although there was a significant decrease among male smokers, there was not as significant a decrease in female smokers.

Athletes use nicotine for a variety of

DRUGS AND ATHLETES

reasons. Some users of tobacco claim that it will cause stimulating effects prior to their athletic performance while others claim that is has calming effects. Some athletes use nicotine for weight reduction.

People who use nicotine may find they have a decreased capacity for work. They also found that smokers have more of a need for oxygen than nonsmokers during exercise. However, others have found no difference in physical work capacity or in oxygen requirements.

When users of nicotine quit using the drug, there is a return of the heart capacity within one day, even with chronic smokers. Therefore, chronic smokers who do not smoke for one day will note an increased improvement in their bodily functions.

Nicotine will stimulate the use of free fatty acids. This will be increased during physical exercise when using nicotine. Smokers are more susceptible to diseases. They also suffer more from inability to sleep than nonsmokers. Therefore, nicotine use can hamper performance in the athlete as lack of sleep would impair physical performance.

Athletes are popularly abusing chewing tobacco. However, chewing tobacco may have similar effects to smoking tobacco.

The Surgeon General warns that cigarette smoking is the leading preventable cause of death in our society. Over 35 years ago, a relation

THE STIMULANTS

between smoking and lung cancer was shown. Lung cancer is now the leading cause of cancer-related deaths in men. Smoking of nicotine will cause an increase in coronary artery disease, heart attacks, and sudden death syndrome. There is also a relationship between nicotine smoking and resultant lung disease. Smoking has caused birth defects in infants and prevented conception in women.

Many types of cancers and dental problems have resulted from the use of chewing tobacco. These cancers were primarily of the mouth and throat. The dental problems include tooth decay, receding of gums and the development of plaque in the mouth. Users of chewing tobacco may also notice an inability to taste and smell.

Nicotine can cause irregular heart beats, convulsions, and toxicity. Nicotine can be addicting. This is shown by users who are unable to stop smoking. Therefore, smoking and chewing of nicotine will significantly affect and trigger heart, lung, oral diseases and cancers. Abstinence is the best therapeutic approach as once someone is addicted to nicotine, either in the form of smoke or "chew", it is difficult to stop.

E. COCAINE

There have been many problems with cocaine abuse among athletes reported in the press. There have been many athletes who have died from cocaine overdose, irregular heart beats, seizures, decreased body temperatures and sudden death syndrome.

DRUGS AND ATHLETES

Feelings of grandeur from cocaine may lead the athlete to believe that he has increased physical and mental abilities. The athlete may feel "high" and stimulated. He may think he is capable of competitive activities that are physically over his limits. This can cause athletic accidents. The athlete can become extremely paranoid which can create problems in athletic competition.

In athletes who abuse cocaine, behavioral differences will be noted. The cocaine abuser may begin to have difficulty with his interpersonal and monetary affairs. He often will not show up for work and will have a tendency to miss assignments. The cocaine user will also become withdrawn. If any of these symptoms are present, it may indicate the abuse of cocaine. (For more information see our book <u>Cocaine: Fact & Fantasy</u>).

IV. <u>CANNABINOIDS</u>

Marijuana, a sedative-hypnotic with mild hallucinogenic properties, is obtained from the top leaves and flowers of the female Indian Hemp plant, Cannabis sativa.

Athletes use marijuana in the same amounts as nonathletes. People who are in the same room as marijuana smokers may show positive for marijuana drug testing. The active ingredient of marijuana is tetrahydrocannabinol (THC). It is taken up very rapidly. Normally, one-half of THC will remain in the body for 5 days. However, due to the fact that it stays in fat cells, THC can remain in the body for up to thirty days.

The athlete who uses marijuana will notice changes in performance ability. Depth perception is altered and may make performing difficult for athletes, particularly in sports like baseball. Time perception is altered, slowing the athlete's response and causing a slow-motion like effect. Memory may be impaired, affecting athletic activities that require complex strategies and coordination.

Athletes may become very paranoid from the side effects of marijuana. This can impair an athlete's ability to perform. Some users of marijuana may also experience hallucinations, which could interfere with an athlete's performance. Marijuana can increase heart rate, pulse rate and cause muscle spasms. These muscle spasms can adversely affect an athlete's performance.

Marijuana can cause a lack of motivation. The user will become withdrawn, unable to complete tasks, easily frustrated, and very apathetic.

The use of marijuana can be, in some situations, extremely dangerous. The alteration in visual depth perception can make operating machinery, driving or performing athletic activities extremely risky. In fact, marijuana can adversely affect driving more than alcohol. Therefore, no benefits have been shown to exist from the use of marijuana by athletes.

V. BETA BLOCKERS

The beta blockers are drugs used primarily for high blood pressure. Beta blockers have also been used therapeutically in the treatment of heart pain, irregular heart beats, anxiety, migraines, and withdrawal. Some of the commonly used beta blockers include propranolol (Inderal), metoprolol (Lopressor), nadolol (Corgard), atenolol (Tenormin), pindolol (Visken) and timolol (Blocadren). The beta-1 receptors are found in the fat tissue, kidneys, and the heart. The beta-2 receptors are found in the arteries, the liver, and the lungs. When the beta receptors are stimulated, this causes stimulation of the heart, widening of the blood vessels, breakdown of fats, breakdown of carbohydrates, and relaxation of smooth muscle in the stomach and lungs.

Most of the beta blockers are beta-1 blocking agents. The drugs will usually have an effect on the heart rate and the fat breakdown. They will usually not have an effect on carbohydrate breakdown or spasms of the lung. However, as the dose of the beta-1 blockers is increased, they will start to block the beta-2 effects.

Athletes frequently abuse beta blockers to decrease their anxiety prior to athletic performance. Lecturers abuse these drugs prior to speaking performances to maintain control and decrease their anxiety. Musicians have used beta blockers to increase their music ability and thereby improve their performance. Athletes in archery and gun shooting are most apt to use these drugs.

BETA BLOCKERS

The problem that athletes encounter when using beta blockers is their adverse effects on energy production. These drugs will interfere with the breakdown of carbohydrates and fats. Athletes competing in endurance sports may have their energy levels adversely affected by using these drugs.

The response to beta blockers in athletes will be variable. The factors that cause the difference in responses include the duration of the medication, the dose of the drug, the timing of the test, and the type of drug administration (oral, intravenous, subcutaneous, etc.). The type of person being studied will also make a dramatic difference (i.e. healthy versus diseased).

The beta blockers can have adverse effects. People with asthma who use beta blockers can develop lung spasms. A decrease in blood pressure, congestive heart failure and slowing of the heart are all effects that can occur. The beta blockers can also affect the central nervous system causing hallucinations and bizarre dreams. Due to the breakdown of carbohydrates, low blood sugar can result. Stomach upset, hair loss, and narrowing of the blood vessels can result from using the beta blockers. Males have noticed sexual impotence while on these medications.

Upon discontinuation of the beta blockers, it is advised to gradually withdraw from these drugs. This is to avoid the symptoms of increased heart rate, tremor, headaches, anxiety, irregular heart beats, and heart pain that may occur.

DRUGS AND ATHLETES

The beta blockers are banned from the Olympic Games in 1988. The primary reason athletes use beta blockers is to prevent anxiety and tremors. However, the combination of adverse effects of beta blockers far outweigh any increased athletic effects the drug may have.

VI. <u>CENTRAL NERVOUS SYSTEM DEPRESSANTS</u>

A. ALCOHOL

Alcohol is used by athletes to decrease anxiety and to obtain relaxation. Alcohol has been an influence in the lives of many athletes. Athletes, who were once believed to avoid alcohol, are now shown to have the same risk of developing alcohol dependency.

Alcohol causes a lowering of inhibitions. It is through this phenomena that athletes may experience an increase in confidence and relaxation prior to an athletic event. Despite their chronic alcohol abuse, many of these athletes have performed extremely effectively. However, there are many side effects that occur with the use of alcohol that far outweigh this performance enhancement.

The use of alcohol will affect the athlete's ability to function accurately. This is an important component in sports including baseball, soccer, archery, and riflery.

The balance of the athlete will also be affected by alcohol abuse. This is an important

THE DEPRESSANTS

component for jumping, which is required in basketball, the high and long jumps, and volleyball. Skating, bicycling and gymnastics also require balance to effectively compete.

An athlete's reaction time can be affected by the use of alcohol. Most sports require quick reaction time for peak performance. Abuse of alcohol can adversely affect hand/eye coordination. Serious injury can occur to athletes when this ability is decreased. The alcohol user will experience interference with motor skills coordination.

Some athletes believe that alcohol may increase muscular strength, although this has not been proven. Alcohol will not cause an increase in endurance. Thus, alcohol does not have an effect on the aerobic capacity of athletes.

High blood pressure can develop with the use of large amounts of alcohol. Lowering of blood pressure may occur with moderate doses of alcohol. Alcoholics have a greater risk of developing coronary artery disease and having a stroke.

Alcohol can stimulate stomach secretions. This can cause inflammation of the stomach, inflammation of the pancreas, and liver damage.

Sexual desire may be increased by alcohol intoxication, but sexual performance may be impaired. Alcohol increases urinary excretion.

Pregnant women who abuse alcohol may

DRUGS AND ATHLETES

cause deformities in the fetus. The mother's alcohol consumption may endanger fetal development, size and nutrition. Newborns may experience withdrawal when born to alcoholic women.

Genetics has been shown to play a key role in predisposing the user to alcohol dependence. Early recognition of alcoholism is important, as alcoholics suffer a myriad of diseases including malnutrition, vitamin deficiency states, inflammation of the liver and heart, fluid imbalances, and skeletal muscle damage.

Vitamin deficiencies may result in alcoholics due to vitamin B deficiency. Neurologically, inability to walk, mental confusion and impaired eye movements may occur.

Alcohol use may also trigger the development of cancer. Cancer of the mouth, digestive tract, lungs, stomach and liver may develop.

The primary effects of alcohol are on thought processes. The alcohol user becomes extroverted and full of confidence. In addition, the use of alcohol may cause emotional swings which are often uncontrolled and can precipitate violence. Initially, physical abilities may appear to be enhanced due to lowering of inhibitions, but as intoxication progresses physical abilities are impaired. An example is the male abusing alcohol who feels like "Casanova" but in reality is unable to maintain an erection.

Alcohol is the number one drug abused in

the United States. Athletes use alcohol for relaxation and anxiety relief. However, alcohol can affect athletic performance through impairment of psychomotor functions. Alcohol affects the regulators of body temperature. Heat loss and low blood sugar can result when an athlete exercises in the cold. Therefore, the overall effect of alcohol on athletic performance is negative.

B. SEDATIVE-HYPNOTICS

The National Institute of Drug Abuse reported that 60% of adults have had a prescription for either a sedative-hypnotic or a mild tranquilizer. The sedative-hypnotics are central nervous system depressants which are prescribed for sleep, anxiety relief, and muscle relaxation. In high doses they are used for epilepsy control, anesthesia and high blood pressure.

Athletes abuse the sedative-hypnotics to relieve anxiety and the stress of competition. However, as with the anti-anxiety drugs, the athlete's performance while using a sedative-hypnotic is impaired. The athlete may have an unrealistic delusion of athletic ability while using sedative-hypnotics. However, the reality is that his physical and psychological performance as an athlete will be impaired.

The adverse effects of the sedative-hypnotics include the potential for heart and lung malfunction, dependency and withdrawal. The athlete will be unable to walk and will appear

DRUGS AND ATHLETES

intoxicated.

An overdose with a sedative-hypnotic can be fatal. The combination of alcohol with a sedative-hypnotic is particularly dangerous as it can increase the toxicity of the sedative-hypnotic.

Drug labels warn that people using sedative-hypnotics or the anti-anxiety drugs should not operate heavy equipment, machinery, or drive an automobile. The reason is that the person abusing the sedative-hypnotic can pose a hazardous situation.

Examples of sedative-hypnotics include the barbiturate agents such as pentobarbital (Nembutal), secobarbital (Seconal), phenobarbital (Luminal), and glutethimide (Doriden).

Sedatives, although they have therapeutic effects, are often abused by people to escape from the stresses of everyday life. Both the sedative-hypnotics and the anti-anxiety agents may impair athletic performance and cause adverse and hazardous side effects.

C. THE BENZODIAZEPINES

The benzodiazepines are mild tranquilizers and anti-anxiety drugs used for depression, muscular tension, alcohol withdrawal and convulsive disorders. Athletes may abuse the benzodiazepine drugs to enable them to cope with stressful situations. Euphoria (a feeling of contentment, well-being and happiness) and

THE DEPRESSANTS

release from reality are other effects which may contribute to abuse potential in athletes. Although the athlete's physical performance will be decreased, he will believe that he is performing at his best. Due to hangover, impaired motor skills, and drowsiness, the athlete's physical and mental abilities can be altered. Users of the benzodiazepines may develop a variety of side effects including headaches, muscular weakness and nausea. This muscular weakness can adversely affect the athlete's physical performance.

The benzodiazepines are used as anti-anxiety drugs. Ironically, with continued use they will cause a disruption of stage four sleep and a resultant increase in anxiety. Sexual function in males and menstruation in females may be impaired.

Discontinuing benzodiazepines after long-term use in high doses will cause a withdrawal syndrome of convulsions, shaking, paranoia, sweating, vomiting, stomach and muscle cramps. This withdrawal syndrome is similar to barbiturate and alcohol withdrawal. Treatment for diazepam (Valium) withdrawal is by gradually decreasing the daily dosage.

Overdose of the benzodiazepines can cause heart and lung malfunction, low blood pressure, confusion and coma.

Examples of the benzodiazepine drugs include diazepam (Valium), chlordiazepoxide (Librium), and flurazepam (Dalmane).

VII. SKELETAL MUSCLE RELAXANTS

Athletic injuries may trigger painful muscle contractions. This is due to the inflammatory response. The muscle relaxants are central nervous system depressants that will interfere with the reflex action.

Muscle spasms are reactions to the inflammatory response. These muscle spasms occur for short periods of time. Therefore, it is difficult to determine the effectiveness of the drug in treating the spasm.

The skeletal muscle relaxants include methocarbomal (Robaxin), orphenadrine citrate (Norflex), carisoprodol (Soma), and cyclobenzaprine (Flexeril). The first effects that occur with these drugs is sedation. They are often combined with other pain medications including aspirin and acetaminophen (Tylenol). The sedative effects may actually cause relief of the muscle spasm. Thus, it is difficult to determine the effectiveness of the skeletal muscle relaxants alone in the treatment of athletic injuries. However, due to the central nervous system depressant effects of these drugs, this can prove a hazardous choice for the athlete.

VIII. PAIN MEDICATIONS

Non-Narcotic Pain Medications

Athletes abuse pain medications (analgesics) to prevent inflammation that occurs with pain. Athletes will often use aspirin at night to prevent the aches and pains that occur from strenuous

PAIN MEDICATIONS

athletic involvement. Of the analgesics, aspirin causes more adverse drug reactions.

Nearly 20,000 tons of aspirin are used annually in the United States. This easy accessability of aspirin has resulted in extensive abuse. Aspirin causes toxic symptoms in ten thousand people in the United States annually. Overuse of aspirin will be indicated by ringing in the ears, nausea, vomiting, and headache. Aspirin can cause other problems including stomach upset, allergic responses and bleeding.

Narcotic Pain Medications

The narcotic pain medications are used for moderate to severe pain. They decrease anxiety and increase the patient's tolerance to pain. Tolerance to the narcotic analgesics develops rapidly and increasingly high doses are needed to obtain the euphoric "high". With prolonged use and in higher doses, the euphoric "high" declines, physical dependence develops, side effects appear and toxic levels may easily be reached.

Some of the narcotic pain medications include: hydromorphone (Dilaudid), oxycodone (used in combination with aspirin to form Percodan and with acetaminophen to formulate Percocet and Tylox), opium (Paregoric), morphine, hydrocodone (Hycodan), codeine, pentazocine (Talwin Nx), propoxyphene (Darvon) and methadone. Athletes use the narcotic analgesics to relieve moderate to severe pain and to eliminate inflammation. The use of the narcotic analgesics masks the protective pain associated

DRUGS AND ATHLETES

with injury, encourages the athlete to continue participation and prevents the initial injury from healing.

IX. <u>ANTI-INFLAMMATORY AGENTS</u>

Athletes often use the nonsteroidal anti-inflammatory drugs to slow the inflammatory response and to alleviate pain from athletic injuries.

One of the most commonly used anti-inflammatory agents is ibuprofen (Advil, Motrin). The side effects of ibuprofen include stomach upset, fluid retention, excess potassium in the blood, and blood diseases. Headaches, dizziness, and ringing of the ears occur with the use of the nonsteroidal anti-inflammatory agents. Bronchial spasms may occur in patients that are allergic to these particular agents. Thus, patients with stomach disorders, liver or kidney ailments, and children or pregnant women should avoid the use of the nonsteroidal anti-inflammatory agents.

X. <u>CORTICOSTEROIDS</u>

Corticosteroids are used by athletes for their ability to reduce inflammation and to cover up the pain that comes with injury. The problem is that it encourages athletes to continue athletic competition which will cause further problems with the initial injury. Corticosteroids are seldom used and have been replaced by the use of the nonsteroidal anti-inflammatory drugs for muscular skeletal problems. Some of the adverse effects of the corticosteroids include the development of brittle bones, high blood pressure, hair growth, inflammation of the pancreas, overgrowth of infections, and inability to heal.

XI. **DIMETHYL SULFOXIDE (DMSO)**

Dimethyl sulfoxide has a unique ability to penetrate skin. Drugs are often combined with DMSO to enhance their topical application and drug effects. DMSO is abused by people to treat musculoskeletal disorders. The adverse effects of DMSO include skin irritation. The safety and efficacy of DMSO has yet to be confirmed and is not approved for use by the Food and Drug Administration.

XII. **BLOOD DOPING**

Athletes use blood doping to increase the oxygen supply to their muscles. This method was used in the 1984 Olympic Games by many athletes prior to competition.

An athlete may remove approximately 1000 milliliters (ml) of his blood and will freeze and store it. After the blood has been drawn, he will supplement his diet with iron and well balanced meals. Immediately prior to competition, the blood will be reinjected into the athlete. The increase of oxygen in the blood may increase the athlete's endurance. However, the increase may be insignificant.

DRUGS AND ATHLETES

Athletes should be aware of the adverse effects that can be incurred from the loss of their own blood or from the use of another person's blood. The body may take weeks or even months to readjust to the blood loss. Other problems can result from the increased thickness of the blood. The surface blood vessel resistance will be increased by raising the blood thickness. The blood can begin to thicken and create health risks. This can result in blood clots which can be fatal.

An athlete who engages in blood doping by using another person's blood may develop many diseases. The primary risk is the development of AIDS, and hepatitis. Inflammation of the heart tissue, serum sickness, and blood incompatibility can also occur. Thus, blood doping has many adverse effects which far outweigh the beneficial effects.

XIII. MISCELLANEOUS DRUGS OF ABUSE

The drugs we have covered in this book are only the most commonly abused drugs in the sports world. There are, however, many other compounds that athletes abuse, prescription, nonprescription and illegal drugs included.

Sodium bicarbonate and potassium citrate are basic substances that decrease the acidity of the blood. In turn, they increase the oxygen-carrying capacity of the blood. The problems that occur with the use of these drugs include severe fluid imbalances and even death.

MISCELLANEOUS DRUGS OF ABUSE

Athletes use the diuretics, which stimulate the flow of urine, for weight loss and dehydration. The dehydration can affect the athlete's performance and may trigger heat injury.

Octacosanol (a solid white alcohol) is abused by athletes to increase strength, endurance, and reaction time. Guarana is an energy booster that has a high caffeine content. It has the same side effects as high doses of caffeine. "Prime Again" is available in pharmacies and athletes use it to increase their testosterone levels. However, two Swedish athletes who used it were suspended for high testosterone levels.

Clomiphene, human chorionic gonadotropin, and tamoxifen (Nolvadex) are used by athletes in high doses to reverse the side effects of the anabolic steroids. Pentoxifylline is used by athletes to help reverse the side effects of blood doping, including increased clotting and excessive blood thickness. Cyproheptadine is abused by athletes to promote weight gain. Gerobital (GH3) is a procaine mixture which has been touted as "the fountain of youth". Athletes abuse this drug for its stimulant effects. Aloe vera is used by athletes to enhance performance, to increase oxygen capacity, and prevent tumors from the abuse of anabolic steroids. However, aloe vera is a potent laxative and will cause the stool to excrete pieces of colon lining tissue. Bee pollen is used by athletes to enhance athletic performance. Athletes believe it will reduce lactic acid in the blood and shorten the recovery time from athletic performance. However, there may be no advantage of using bee pollen.

DRUGS AND ATHLETES

Gensing is used by athletes for anabolic effects although this has not been proven.

Proteolytic enzymes, which breakdown proteins like papain, are used by athletes to control inflammation from injury. However, they will impair the absorption of the antibiotic agents. Vitamin B15 (Pangamic acid) is abused by athletes to keep their muscle tissue operating at a peak capacity. However, 90% of the athletes who take this drug assume the risk of developing liver cancer within seven years. Amino acids, including combinations of arginine and ornithine, are nutritional supplements that are used by athletes. However, they do have high nitrogen contents and can thereby damage the kidney.

As previously discussed, there are a whole array of drugs that are abused by athletes. We have covered just a few in this course. (For further information see <u>Drugs of Abuse</u> and <u>Cocaine: Fact and Fantasy</u>.)

XIV. <u>DRUG CONTROL PROGRAMS OF THE OLYMPIC COMMITTEE</u>

Widespread drug abuse in athletics between 1950 and 1970 led to eventual laboratory testing for drug abuse. In 1960, at the Rome Olympics, a Danish cyclist abused stimulants and died. A Tour De France contestant died while using amphetamines. Olympic physicians demanded action when athletes at the games in Tokyo, 1964, indicated a high degree of drug abuse. In 1965, France and Belgium passed anti-doping laws. The

TABLE I

SUBSTANCES BANNED BY THE INTERNATIONAL OLYMPIC COMMITTEE

I. <u>Anabolic Steroids</u>
clostebol, dehydrochlormethyltestosterone, fluoxymesterone, mesterolone, methenolone, methandienone, methyltestosterone, nandrolone, norethandrolone, oxymesterone, oxymetholone, stanozolol, testosterone* and related compounds

II. <u>Psychomotor Stimulant Drugs</u>
amphetamine, benzphetamine, chlorphentermine, cocaine, diethylpropion, dimethylamphetamine, ethylamphetamine, fencamfamin, meclofenoxate, methylamphetamine, methylphenidate, norpseudoephedrine, pemoline, phendimetrazine, phenmetrazine, phentermine, pipradol, prolintane, and related compounds

III. <u>Sympathomimetic Amines</u>
chlorprenaline, ephedrine, etafedrine, isoetharine, isoprenaline, methoxyphenamine, methylephedrine, and related compounds

IV. <u>Narcotic Analgesics</u>
anileridine, codeine, dextromoramide, dihydrocodeine, dipipanone, ethylmorphine, heroin, hydrocodone, hydromorphone, levorphanol, methadone, morphine, oxomorphone, pentazocine, pethidinephenazocine, piminodine, thebacon, trimeperidine, and related compounds

V. <u>Miscellaneous Central Nervous System Stimulants</u>
amiphenazole, bemigride, caffeine*, cropropamide

DRUGS AND ATHLETES

(component of "micoren"), crotethamide (component of "micoren"), doxapram, ethamivan, leptazol, nikethamide

---

At the request of the International Federations (F.I.E. and U.I.P.M.B.), an alcohol test will be performed during competitions.

*Definition of positive depends on the following: For caffeine: if the concentration in urine exceeds 15 micrograms/ml. For testosterone: if the ration of the total concentration of testosterone to that of epitestosterone in the urine exceeds 6.

European Council defined doping as "the administering or use of substances in any form alien to the body or of physiological substances in abnormal amounts and with abnormal methods by healthy persons with the exclusive aim of obtaining an artificial and unfair increase of performance and competition." In 1967, the International Olympic Committee (IOC) established the medical commission for doping control.

In 1965, gas chromatography (GC) was used to test for drugs. GC is now combined with mass spectrometry (MS) to test for doping control. All International Sports Federations as of 1972 have required this combination drug testing identification. It was not until 1976 that it was possible to effectively test an athlete for anabolic steroids. In 1976, the IOC added anabolic steroids to their list of banned substances. In 1984, the Olympic Games in Los Angeles utilized GC/MS drug analysis for anabolic steroids in all contestants.

OLYMPIC DRUG CONTROL PROGRAMS

There are many factors that can influence how long a drug will stay in a person's system and continue to be detected. The factors that have to be considered are the dose, the drug formulation, the route of administration, the breakdown of drugs in the body, alterations in the body's functions (including disease states), and the detection factors used in drug testing.

There are five different categories of drugs considered doping agents by the Olympic Committee (see Chart I). Athletes who are discovered to have these drugs in their system prior to an athletic performance are disqualified from the game.

XV. **IDENTIFYING THE DRUG ABUSER**

It is difficult to determine whether a person has a chemical dependency problem. There are symptoms, behavioral and physical, that may indicate a drug abuse problem.

The first thing to look for is obvious intoxication or for the smell of marijuana or alcohol. The person's physical appearance may be altered, becoming extremely unkempt. The personality will change with dramatic mood swings. The person will become dishonest. The drug abuser may be arrested for problems with the law. He may appear to be depressed a great amount of the time. His relationships with others will begin to deteriorate. The person will become reclusive and will begin to change the people that he associates with.

DRUGS AND ATHLETES

If the drug abuser is a student, his grades will decline, he will fail to show up at school, and will fail to observe curfew and to attend to household chores. The adult will frequently change or lose his job. The drug abuser will begin withdrawing from all outside activities. He will lose interest in recreational activities. Money and other items may be missing as the drug abuser continues to channel these to support his drug habit.

When someone tries to talk to the drug abuser about drugs, he will quickly change the subject and refuse to discuss it. This is the most difficult thing, attempting to get the drug abuser to admit that he has a drug related problem. The drug abuser will hide his drugs, alcohol or drug paraphernalia secretly. This is to avoid his fear of being "found out". It is important to try to recognize and treat the drug abuser in the early stages if possible.

XVI. <u>CASE STUDIES</u>

CASE I

A female bodybuilder began using anabolic steroids to stimulate her physique, believing that the steroid drugs would help her develop larger muscles and stimulate the muscle building properties. She also hoped that the steroid effects would enable her to get to the top of her profession. She did indeed win many contests and became rated as the top amateur female bodybuilder in the world.

CASE STUDIES

However, the drugs began making her develop masculine characteristics. She grew facial hair and her muscles began to bulge. Her voice became very deep and her breast tissue was eliminated. The drugs also made her extremely aggressive and antagonistic. She was very depressed.

The anabolic steroids did increase her strength and her weightlifting ability. Her muscles became very large. She did indeed win many body building contests throughout the world as a result of her anabolic steroid abuse. However, the side effects that she endured from the drugs far outweighed any positive benefits she had gained.

CASE II

On June 17, 1987, Len Bias, a 22-year-old University of Maryland basketball star, began celebrating his selection as a member of the Boston Celtics basketball team. This celebration unfortunately ended with his death, which was due to cocaine intoxication. Previously, literature had reported that cocaine use could cause death from heart damage.

In Bias's autopsy report, the microscopic sections of the heart stated "additional sections of right and left ventricular myocardium reveal tiny foci of lymphocytic macrophage infiltrate and in one left ventricular section there is evidence of fibrin necrosis." A cocaine induced toxic heart disorder is the condition that was responsible for this alteration in the heart.

DRUGS AND ATHLETES

The autopsy report also stated "all lobes of both lungs appear diffusely congested and on sectioning there is a copious amount of edema fluid with a large amount of white frothy edema fluid present in the lumen of the trachea and both mainstem bronchi." Cocaine in large doses can cause fast, irregular and very shallow breathing.

Cocaine was found in Len Bias's body; 6.5 mg. per liter in the heart blood, 63 mg. per liter in the bile, and 12 mg. per kilogram in the kidney.

Thus, the chief medical examiner determined that Len Bias "died as a result of cocaine intoxication, which interrupted the normal electrical control of his heart beat, resulting in the sudden onset of seizures and cardiac arrest."

Thus, cocaine can cause sudden heart death syndromes. This may occur in people who exercise strenuously. The stimulation of norepinephrine from exercising and cocaine will stimulate the effects of cocaine. Cocaine can cause increased heart rate, high blood pressure, heart attacks, and as in the case of Len Bias, sudden cardiac death. Twenty milligrams of cocaine can be fatal, although most journals estimate that a dose of 1200 mg. intravenously is the normal toxic dose.

CASE III

Don Rogers, a defensive back for the Cleveland Browns football team, died on June 27, 1986. The 23-year-old Rogers was to have been

CASE STUDIES

married the following day. Just like Len Bias, Rogers was not known to have been a drug abuser. Rogers attended a bachelor party in his honor. The following morning he began "feeling funny" and was rushed to the emergency department in Sacramento, California when he began having convulsions and jerking movements. Upon his arrival at the emergency room his pupils were dilated, his pulse had ceased, and no other responses were seen. He was immediately transferred to another hospital to undergo resuscitation measures. However, he died nearly five hours later.

The autopsy report indicated that the blood was positive for cocaine and was at a lethal level. The brain had 10 mg per kg of cocaine, the lung had 7.3 mg per kg, and the kidney had 4.5 mg per kg. The cause of death reported on the autopsy was severe congestion and swelling in the lungs which was caused by cocaine intoxication.

The Cleveland Browns have developed an aggressive security program to prevent drug dealers from mingling with the players. Their drug treatment program, "Inner Circle", has been in existence for six years and focuses on aftercare.

CASE IV

A 24-year-old male power-lifter was admitted to a hospital in December of 1980, when after attempting to lift 750 pounds, his knees gave out and he had collapsed on the ground. Afterwards, he was having difficulty walking. The athlete

DRUGS AND ATHLETES

was discovered to have a rupture of his left leg and a minor rupture of his right arm. The patient recovered following surgery and returned to compete as a heavyweight power-lifter.

The athlete was determined to have taken numerous drugs. This included methandrostenolone (Dianabol), testosterone intramuscularly twice a week and chorionic gonadotropin. These drugs were taken for 2 1/2 months prior to the athletic event. The day before the athletic event the athlete also took a diuretic agent, furosemide (Lasix) intramuscularly and orally. The athlete also ingested potassium orally and 16 tablets of sodium chloride. Due to the effects of the diuretic, the athlete lost over 10 pounds.

Multiple drug abuse problems also occur in athletes. This case demonstrates that athletes are abusing anabolic steroids and a variety of drug combinations without medical supervision.

XVII. <u>CONCLUSION</u>

Anyone supervising athletes should not recommend or prescribe drugs to enhance their performance. This behavior is a violation of professional ethics for health practitioners. The American College of Sports Medicine stated in 1977 that "serious continuing efforts should be made to educate male and female athletes, coaches, physical educators, physicians, trainers and the general public regarding the inconsistent effects of anabolic steroids on improvement of human physical performance and the potential

CONCLUSION

danger of taking certain forms of these substances, especially in large doses for prolonged periods."

Athletes need to be educated regarding the adverse effects and potential toxicity of the drugs being abused in the sports world. They should not experiment with drugs which they know nothing about. Athletes may lack the will and determination to change their athletic abilities through exercising and inner strength. Instead they seek support with drugs.

Drug misuse and abuse are not unique or new to our culture. Athletes are also influenced by the social acceptance of drugs in society. The legal ramifications of drug abuse have done little to stem the tide of drugs. People look to athletes as leaders and role models. Their influence on our society and our children is astounding.

Drugs most commonly abused by athletes are nicotine, alcohol, marijuana and cocaine. Addiction by athletes to all drugs is seen more frequently.

The image of sports has been plagued with a history of drug abuse. Athletes abuse these drugs for performance enhancement, relaxation, celebration, or to prevent physical or mental pain.

Athletes who abuse drugs to achieve a winning performance, may have unknown side effects from the drugs. They may also trade a short term gain for a very long term drug problem.

BIBLIOGRAPHY

1. Steroids in Sports, "After Four Decades Time To Return These Genies To Bottle?" Med News/Persp, Jan 23-30,1987, 2574, 421-426.
2. "Illicit Drugs and the Athlete," Am Phar Jrnl, Vol NS 26,#11, Nov 86;9-42.
3. Birdsong, Carl, "Why Athletes Use Drugs," American Pharmacy Journal, Vol. NS26, #11, Nov 1986, 43-45.
4. Bertacchi, G., Cocaine: Fact & Fantasy, NMS, October 1987.
5. Bertacchi, G., Drugs of Abuse, NMS, Dec 1986.
6. Hill, J.A., Suker, J.R., Sachs, K., Brigham, C., "The Athletic Polydrug Abuse Phenomenon. A Case Report," Am J Sports Med, Jul-Aug 1983;29(3):221-3.7.
7. Murray, T.H., "The Coercive Power of Drugs in Sports," Hasting Cent Rep, Aug 1983;13(4):24-30.
8. Haupt, H.A.; Rovere, G.D., "Anabolic Steroids: A Review of the Literature," Am J Sports Med Nov-Dec 1984; 12(6):469-84.
9. Ryan, A.J., "Causes and Remedies for Drug Misuse and Abuse by Athletes," JAMA Jul 1984, 27;252(4):517-9.
10. Cowart,"Physician-Competitor's Advice to Colleag:Steroid Users Respond to Education, Rehab (news),"JAMA,Jan'87,23-30;257(4):427-8.
11. Perlmutter, G., "Use of Anabolic Steroids by Athletes," Am Fam Physician, Oct 1985;32(4):208-10.
12. Beckett, A.H., "Sports Injuries. Drugs in Sports," British Journal of Hospital Medicine, March 1983,29(3):221-3.
13. Lamb, David R., "Anabolic Steroids in Athletics: How Well Do They Work and How Dangerous Are They?" American Journal of Sports Medicine, Jan-Feb 1984,12(1):31-8.
14. Oseid, Svein, "Doping & Athletes-Prevention & Counseling," Jour of Aller and Clin Immun, May 1984, 73(5PT2):735-9.
15. Delbeke, F. T., and Debackere, M., "Caffeine: Use and Abuse in Sports," Int J. Sports Med, Aug; 1984, 5(4):10-5.
16. "Drugs in the Olympics," Medical Letter Drugs Therapeutics, July 6, 1984; 26(665):65-6.
17. Catlin, D.H., et al., "Analyt Chem at Games of the 23rd Olympiad in LA, 1984," Clin Chem 1987 Feb; 33 (2P+1):319-27.

GLOSSARY

ABSTINENCE- Self-denial, usually voluntary refraining from taking drugs, sex or alcohol.

ADVERSE EFFECTS- A side effect produced by a drug other than the one sought.

AIDS- Acquired Immune Deficiency Syndrome; a deadly disease that impairs one's immune system and has almost a 100% death rate within 3 years of diagnosis.

ALKALOID- Any one of a class of compounds which forms salts with acids and soaps with fats.

ANABOLIC STEROIDS- Drugs derived from the male hormone testosterone abused by athletes to increase athletic prowess.

ANALGESIC- A pain medication.

ANEMIA- A condition in which blood is deficient in quantity, in red cells, or in hemoglobin and which is marked by pallor, weakness, and irregular heart action.

ANESTHESIA- Loss of sensation, induced from a drug prior to surgery.

APATHETIC- Lack of interest or emotion.

ARTERIES- A vessel that carries blood away from the heart.

AUTOPSY- The examination of a dead body to determine the cause of death.

BENZODIAZEPINES- Drugs that are classified as anti-anxiety agents.

BETA BLOCKERS- Drugs used for high blood pressure, heart pain, anxiety, migraines, and withdrawal.

BIRTH DEFECTS- A physical or mental handicap that one is born with.

BLOOD CYST DISORDERS- A number of blood diseases that cause growths of cells.

CAFFEINISM- The state caused by the adverse effects of caffeine.

GLOSSARY

CARBOHYDRATES- A sugar or starch.
CANCER- A tumor that tends to spread throughout the body and often causes death.
CHRONIC SMOKER- One who smokes cigarettes habitually.
CLITORIS- A small erectile organ at the forward part of the vulva of the female.
CONCEPTION- The action of becoming pregnant in the womb.
CONGESTION- An obstruction or blockage in the body.
CONVULSIONS- Violent, involuntary contracting and relaxing of the muscles.
CORONARY ARTERY DISEASE- When the arteries supplying the heart become narrow or clotted causing damage to the heart muscle.
CYST- A sore containing fluid, blood, secretions, etc.
DEPENDENCY- A state characterized by an addiction to a drug which will cause withdrawal if it is discontinued.
DIGESTIVE TRACT- The region in which food travels through to be broken down and digested.
DIURETIC- A drug that increases the flow of urine.
EDEMA FLUID- A watery fluid that accumulates and causes swelling in the tissues or cavities of the body.
ESTROGEN- One of three hormones produced in female ovaries that cause a series of mental changes in females, especially in the reproductive or sexual organs.
EUPHORIA- A feeling of happiness, bodily well-being, and contentment.
FATAL- Deadly.
FATIGUE- Tiredness.

GLOSSARY

FATTY ACIDS- An acid originating from the element called hydrocarbon.

FATTY TISSUE- Provides a reserve supply of energy.

FIBRIN NECROSIS- When a body protein hardens and causes tissue death.

GONADOTROPIN- A substance which has a stimulating effect upon the gonads, especially the hormone secreted by the pituitary.

GRANDEUR- A feeling of greatness.

HALF-LIFE- The time it takes for half of a drug to be eliminated from the body.

HALLUCINATION- A seeing or hearing of things that have no basis outside one's brain.

HEPATITIS- Viral inflammation of the liver.

HORMONES- A chemical substance produced in the body which has a specific effect on the activity of a certain organ(s).

HYPOTHALAMUS- The part of the brain below the higher brain center.

IBUPROFEN- An anti-inflammatory drug used in the treatment of arthritis.

INFLAMMATION- The reaction of tissue to injury, manifested by pain, heat, swelling, and redness.

INTESTINE- The part of the digestive tract from the stomach to the anus.

INTOXICATION- A state of drunkenness.

INTRAMUSCULARLY- Into the muscles.

INTRAVENOUS- Into the veins.

LIVER TUMORS- A swelling or growth on the liver.

LOW BLOOD SUGAR- The opposite of diabetes, a pre-diabetic condition.

LUMEN- The space within a tubular organ, as in a blood vessel.

GLOSSARY

MAINSTEM BRONCHI- The main air passageway of the lungs.
MENSTRUATION- A discharge of body fluid from the womb of the female occurring approximately every four weeks.
METABOLISM- The process of breakdown into basic elements.
METABOLIC RATE-
MUSCLE SPASM- A sudden, abnormal, involuntary contraction of a muscle.
MUSCULOSKELETAL SYSTEM- The bones, muscles, ligaments, tendons, and joints.
NOREPINEPHRINE- A hormone produced in the brain that is used to treat low blood pressure and shock.
PANCREAS- A gland near the stomach that discharges fluid into the intestine to help digestion.
PAPAIN- An enzyme that aids in the digestion of protein.
PITUITARY GLAND- The endocrine gland located at the base of the brain responsible for regulating growth.
PLAQUE- A deposit on the teeth.
PREMENSTRUAL TENSION- A period of tension, irritability, headache, swelling and pain in the breasts, seen in women a few days before menstruation.
PROTEIN SYNTHESIS- The formation of protein out of simple substances.
PSYCHOMOTOR FUNCTIONS- Of or designating muscular activity directly related to mental processes.
RAPID EYE MOVEMENT SLEEP- The period of sleep during which the brain waves are fast and dreaming occurs.

GLOSSARY

RESUSCITATION- The bringing back of a person to life or consciousness.

SEDATION- The state of being calm, relaxed or free from excitement.

SEDATIVE-HYPNOTIC- A drug given to calm the nerves and produce sleep.

SEIZURES- A sudden convulsion.

SERUM SICKNESS- An illness following the injection of the serum into an allergic person.

SIDE EFFECTS- An adverse effect produced by a drug other than the one sought.

STIMULANTS- Any drug that temporarily increases the activity of some part of the body.

STROKE- The sudden rupture or clotting of a blood vessel to the brain.

SUDDEN DEATH SYNDROME- The quick death of an individual, most commonly triggered by a drug reaction which causes heart failure.

SYNTHETIC PRODUCT- A product that does not occur naturally but is man-made.

TENDONS- Cords of connective tissue that attach muscle to bone or cartilage.

TESTES- The reproductive organs in the male where sperm is developed.

TESTOSTERONE- The male sex hormone, manufactured and secreted by the testicles.

TISSUE- An aggregation of cells that are similar in type.

TRACHEA- The air breathing tube between the mouth and lungs.

TRANQUILIZERS- A large class of drugs used to treat anxiety and mental disorders.

TRANSSEXUAL- A person (male or female) who undergoes a sex change operation to become a member of the opposite sex.

GLOSSARY

ULCER- A lesion or open sore that occurs on the surface of any organ or tissue.
VENTRICULAR MYOCARDIUM- The heart muscle cavity.

GENERAL PUBLIC BOOKS
REGISTRATION FORM (Please Print or Type)

NATIONAL MEDICAL SEMINARS, INC.
P.O. BOX 2699; ROSEVILLE, CA 95746
US (800) 331-8777 LOCAL (916) 784-6200
CA (800) 331-4747 FAX (916) 784-3979

Name_____

Address_____

City_____State_____Zip_____

Home Phone (_____)_____

Work Phone (_____)_____

Please send me the following General Public books:

____	Book #1 Aids, Sex, and Protection	$4.95
____	Book #2 Athletes and Drugs	$4.95
____	Book #3 Birth Control Choices	$4.95
____	Book #4 Cocaine: Fact and Fantasy	$4.95
____	Book #5 Diet Secrets for Weight Control	$4.95
____	Book #6 Drugs of Abuse	$4.95
____	Book #7 Drugs, Sex, and Aging	$4.95
____	Book #8 Pregnancy Care	$4.95
____	Book #9 Hawaiian Heat	$4.95

<u>First Class Postage & Handling (per book)</u>..................................$1.00
(In California add 6% sales tax)

____ Enclosed is my check or money order

MC, VISA, AE #_____

Credit Card Expiration Date_____

Signature_____